The Complete Low Cholesterol Cookbook For Beginners UK

Nourishing Your Heart: Delicious and Nutritious Recipes for a Healthy Heart Journey, 3200 Days of superb Recipes, With a 31 Days Meal Plan.

Wilbur Avery

Table Of Contents

INTRODUCTION

Introducing Janet, a health-conscious person determined to put her heart health first. Janet recognizes the value of sticking to a low-cholesterol diet in a world where convenience and quick food are frequently prioritised. For this reason, she consults "The Complete Low Cholesterol Cookbook For Beginners UK," her reliable traveling companion in the kitchen.

This cookbook is not your average compilation of recipes; rather, it is an extensive manual designed especially for these new to heart-healthy living in the United Kingdom. We explore a world of tasty recipes meant to control cholesterol levels without sacrificing flavor, with Janet as our guide.

Janet finds a wealth of 2800 days' worth of dishes in the pages of this cookbook, guaranteeing a varied and fascinating culinary adventure. Every meal, from delectable breakfast selections to beautiful lunches, filling dinners, and even tantalizing desserts, is skillfully prepared to support heart health.

Janet is overjoyed to discover a variety of dishes using easily accessible, locally sourced, fresh foods in the UK. She learns how to lower cholesterol intake without sacrificing the enjoyment of food through creative cooking methods, astute ingredient swaps, and practical advice.

Janet discovers this cookbook is more than just a collection of recipes as she turns the pages. It serves as an instructional tool, giving her important facts about cholesterol, its effects on health, and the actions she may take to keep her diet wholesome and well-balanced.

Equipped with this newfound knowledge and a plethora of mouthwatering meals, Janet sets off on her low-cholesterol path with confidence and enthusiasm. She is aware that every meal she cooks from "The Complete Low Cholesterol Cookbook For Beginners UK" moves her one step closer to having a heart that is healthier and happier.

Come along with Janet as she shares, one delicious recipe at a time, the keys to a satisfying low-cholesterol lifestyle. Allow this cookbook to serve as your reliable guide as you embark on your personal road to a heart-healthy, vibrant future.

Our bodies' cells contain the waxy, fat-like material known as cholesterol. High cholesterol, especially low-density lipoprotein (LDL) cholesterol, can raise the risk of heart disease even though it is necessary for many body processes.

Making educated judgments regarding our nutrition and lifestyle requires an understanding of the relationship between heart health and cholesterol levels. Elevated low-density lipoprotein (LDL) cholesterol can cause plaque to accumulate in the arteries, narrowing them and limiting heart-lung blood flow. Serious illnesses like coronary artery disease, heart attacks, and strokes may arise from this.

Remember that not all cholesterol is harmful. Known as "good" cholesterol, high-density lipoprotein (HDL) cholesterol helps keep arteries and the bloodstream free of excess low-density lipoprotein (LDL) cholesterol.

High cholesterol is caused by a number of things, such as obesity, smoking, a poor diet high in saturated and trans fats, inactivity, and specific medical disorders. Cholesterol levels can also be influenced by genetics.

Living a heart-healthy lifestyle is essential to maintaining a healthy cholesterol profile. This entails eating a well-balanced diet reduced in sodium, cholesterol, and saturated and trans fats. Rather, concentrate on including high-fiber foods like fruits, vegetables, whole grains, and legumes. Keeping a healthy weight, controlling stress, exercising frequently, and quitting smoking are all essential for preserving ideal heart health.

It is advised that people get regular cholesterol screenings, particularly if they have other risk factors or a family history of heart disease. Through the monitoring of cholesterol levels, people can collaborate with medical professionals to create customized plans for controlling cholesterol and lowering the risk of heart disease.

Being aware of heart health issues and cholesterol allows us to take preventative measures for our cardiovascular health. Making educated decisions regarding our food, way of life, and medical care will help us work toward a healthier future and lower our chance of developing heart-related problems.

CHAPTER ONE

Recipes for Breakfast

Light and Airy Oatmeal Pancakes!

Recipe 1:

Light and Airy Oatmeal Pancakes

Information about Nutrition:
- 220 calories
- 7g of total fat
- 2g of saturated fat
- 60 mg of cholesterol
- 400 mg of sodium
- 33g of carbohydrates
- 4g of fiber
- 6g of sugars
- 8g of protein

20 minutes for cooking
Four pancakes are served.

Components:
- One cup of traditional oats
– One cup flour, whole wheat
– Two tsp of brown sugar
- One tablespoon of powdered sugar
- One-half teaspoon of salt

- One cup of milk (or, for a dairy-free option, plant-based milk)
- One-half cup Greek yogurt, plain
- Two sizable eggs
- One tsp of vanilla extract
- Greasing the pan with melted butter or cooking spray

Guidelines:
1. Pulse the oats in a food processor or blender until they resemble flour.
2. Mix the oat flour, whole wheat flour, brown sugar, baking powder, and salt together in a large mixing bowl. Blend thoroughly.
3. Mix the milk, Greek yogurt, eggs, and vanilla extract thoroughly in a another bowl.
4. Mixing until just mixed, pour the wet components into the dry ingredients. It's alright to have a few lumps; don't overmix.
5. Heat a griddle or nonstick skillet to medium. Apply a thin layer of melted butter or cooking spray to the surface.
6. Using the back of a spoon, gently spread 1/4 cup amounts of batter onto the skillet to create a spherical shape.
7. Cook until golden brown, about 2 to 3 minutes per side for the pancakes. Carefully flip with a spatula.
8. Grease the pan if necessary, then repeat the process with the remaining batter.
9. Warm fluffy oatmeal pancakes can be served with sliced bananas, fresh berries, or a honey drizzle as toppings.

Recipe 2:

Traditional Fuffy Oatmeal Pancakes

Per-serving Nutritional Information:
- 220 calories
- 7g of total fat
- 2g of saturated fat
- 60 mg of cholesterol
- 400 mg of sodium

- 33g of carbohydrates
- 4g of fiber
- 6g of sugars
- 8g of protein

20 minutes for cooking
Two pancakes are served.

Components:
- One cup of traditional oats
- One cup flour (all-purpose)
– Two tsp of brown sugar
- Two tsp powdered baking
- One-half teaspoon of salt
- One cup of milk
- 1/4 cup of applesauce without sugar
- Two sizable eggs
- One tsp of vanilla extract
- Greasing the pan with melted butter or cooking spray

Guidelines:
1. Grind the oats in a food processor or blender to a fine texture similar to flour.
2. Mix the brown sugar, baking powder, oat flour, all-purpose flour, and salt together in a mixing dish. Blend thoroughly.
3. Mix the eggs, vanilla essence, applesauce, and milk thoroughly in a another bowl.
4. Mixing until just mixed, pour the wet components into the dry ingredients. It's alright to have a few lumps; don't overmix.
5. Heat a griddle or nonstick skillet to medium. Apply a thin layer of melted butter or cooking spray to the surface.
6. Transfer 1/4 cup sections of batter into the skillet, forming it into a circular shape by gently spreading it with the back of a spoon.
7. Cook until golden brown, about 2 to 3 minutes per side for the pancakes. Carefully flip with a spatula.

8. Grease the pan if necessary, then repeat the process with the remaining batter.

9. Warm up these fluffy oatmeal pancakes and top with your preferred toppings, like Greek yogurt, fresh fruit, or maple syrup.

Recipe 3:

Oatmeal Pancakes with Blueberries

Per-serving Nutritional Information:
- 250 calories
- 8g of total fat
- 2g of saturated fat
- 65 mg of cholesterol
- 400 mg of sodium
- 38g of carbohydrates
- 5g of fiber
- 9g of sugars
- 9g of protein

25 minutes for cooking
Two pancakes are served.

Components:
- One cup of traditional oats
– One cup flour, whole wheat
– Two tsp of brown sugar
- Two tsp powdered baking
- One-half teaspoon of cinnamon
- One-fourth teaspoon of salt
- One cup of milk
- 1/4 cup of applesauce without sugar
- Two sizable eggs
- One tsp of vanilla extract
- A single cup of blueberries

- Greasing the pan with melted butter or cooking spray

Guidelines:
1. Pulse the oats in a food processor or blender until they are finely ground and resemble flour.
2. Mix together the oat flour, whole wheat flour, brown sugar, cinnamon, baking powder, and salt in a mixing dish. Blend thoroughly.
3. Mix the eggs, vanilla essence, applesauce, and milk thoroughly in a another bowl.
4. Mixing until just mixed, pour the wet components into the dry ingredients. Add the fresh blueberries and fold gently.
5. Heat a griddle or nonstick skillet to medium. Apply a thin layer of melted butter or cooking spray to the surface.
6. Transfer 1/4 cup sections of batter into the skillet, forming it into a circular shape by gently spreading it with the back of a spoon.
7. Cook until golden brown, about 2 to 3 minutes per side for the pancakes. Carefully flip with a spatula.
8. Grease the pan if necessary, then repeat the process with the remaining batter.
9. Garnish the warm blueberry oatmeal pancakes with extra blueberries, powdered sugar, or a honey drizzle.

Recipe 4:

Pancakes with Chocolate Chip Oatmeal

Per-serving Nutritional Information:
- There are 290 calories.
- 11g of total fat
- 3g of saturated fat
- 60 mg of cholesterol
- 400 mg of sodium
- 39g of carbohydrates
- 4g of fiber
- 10g of sugars

- 9g of protein

25 minutes for cooking
Two pancakes are served.

Components:
- One cup of traditional oats
- One cup flour (all-purpose)
– Two tsp of brown sugar
- Two tsp powdered baking
- One-half teaspoon of cinnamon
- One-fourth teaspoon of salt
- One cup of milk
- 1/4 cup of applesauce without sugar
- Two sizable eggs
- One tsp of vanilla extract
- Half a cup of chocolate chips
- Greasing the pan with melted butter or cooking spray

Guidelines:
1. Grind the oats in a food processor or blender to a fine texture similar to flour.
2. Mix together the brown sugar, oat flour, all-purpose flour, baking powder, cinnamon, and salt in a mixing dish. Blend thoroughly.
3. Mix the eggs, vanilla essence, applesauce, and milk thoroughly in a another bowl.
4. Mixing until just mixed, pour the wet components into the dry ingredients. It's alright to have a few lumps; don't overmix.
5. Add the chocolate chunks and fold gently.
6. Heat a griddle or nonstick skillet to medium. Apply a thin layer of melted butter or cooking spray to the surface.
7. Transfer 1/4 cup sections of batter into the skillet, forming it into a circular shape by gently spreading it with the back of a spoon.
8. Cook until golden brown, about 2 to 3 minutes per side for the pancakes. Carefully flip with a spatula.

9. Grease the pan if necessary, then repeat the process with the remaining batter.

10. Drizzle some maple syrup and add some extra chocolate chips to the steaming chocolate chip oatmeal pancakes.

Recipe 5:

Pancakes with Apple Cinnamon Oatmeal

Per-serving Nutritional Information:
- 260 calories
- 7g of total fat
- 2g of saturated fat
- 60 mg of cholesterol
- 400 mg of sodium
- 42g of carbohydrates
- 5g of fiber
- 12g of sugars
- 8g of protein

25 minutes for cooking
Two pancakes are served.

Components:
- One cup of traditional oats
- One cup flour (all-purpose)
– Two tsp of brown sugar
- Two tsp powdered baking
- One-half teaspoon of cinnamon
- One-fourth teaspoon of salt
- One cup of milk
- 1/4 cup of applesauce without sugar
- Two sizable eggs
- One tsp of vanilla extract
- One apple, cored, peeled, and diced finely

- Greasing the pan with melted butter or cooking spray

Guidelines:
1. Grind the oats in a food processor or blender to a fine texture similar to flour.
2. Mix together the brown sugar, oat flour, all-purpose flour, baking powder, cinnamon, and salt in a mixing dish. Blend thoroughly.
3. Mix the eggs, vanilla essence, applesauce, and milk thoroughly in a another bowl.
4. Mixing until just mixed, pour the wet components into the dry ingredients. It's alright to have a few lumps; don't overmix.
5. Add the chopped apple and fold gently.
6. Heat a griddle or nonstick skillet to medium. Apply a thin layer of melted butter or cooking spray to the surface.
7. Transfer 1/4 cup sections of batter into the skillet, forming it into a circular shape by gently spreading it with the back of a spoon.
8. Cook until golden brown, about 2 to 3 minutes per side for the pancakes. Carefully flip with a spatula.
9. Grease the pan if necessary, then repeat the process with the remaining batter.
10. Warm apple cinnamon oatmeal pancakes should be served warm with a drizzle of maple syrup or honey and a dusting of cinnamon.

Egg White Scramble with Veggies

Recipe 1:

Egg White Scramble with Spinach and Mushroom Veggie

Per-serving Nutritional Information:
- 180 calories
- 6g of total fat
- 1g of saturated fat
- There is no cholesterol.

- 350 mg of sodium
- 10g of carbohydrates
- 4g of fiber
- 4g of sugars
20g of protein

15 minutes for cooking
Serving Dimensions: 1

Components:
- One teaspoon of extra virgin olive oil
- 1/4 cup of mushroom slices
- One cup of raw spinach
- Egg whites, 3/4 cup (about 6 big egg whites)
To taste, add salt and pepper.

Guidelines:
1. In a nonstick skillet, warm the olive oil over medium heat.
2. When the mushrooms begin to soften, add the slices and sauté for two to three minutes.
3. Cook the fresh spinach leaves in the skillet for a further one to two minutes, or until they have wilted.
4. Add salt and pepper to taste and pour the egg whites into the skillet.
5. Gently stir the mixture and heat for 3–4 minutes, or until the egg whites are scrambled and cooked through.
6. After turning off the heat, move the scramble to a platter.
7. Enjoy and warm up!

Recipe 2:

Vegetable Egg White Scramble with Bell Pepper and Onion

Per-serving Nutritional Information:
- 160 calories
- 5g of total fat

- 1g of saturated fat
- There is no cholesterol.
- 300 milligrams of sodium
- 12g of carbohydrates
- 3g of fiber
- 6g of sugars
- 18g of protein

20 minutes for cooking
Serving Dimensions: 1

Components:
- One teaspoon of extra virgin olive oil
- 1/4 cup of red bell pepper, chopped
Diced green bell pepper, 1/4 cup
1/4 cup finely chopped onion
- Egg whites, 3/4 cup (about 6 big egg whites)
To taste, add salt and pepper.

Guidelines:
1. In a nonstick skillet, warm the olive oil over medium heat.
2. Add the onion and bell peppers that have been diced to the skillet and cook for 4–5 minutes, or until they are soft.
3. Add salt and pepper to taste and pour the egg whites into the skillet.
4. Gently stir the mixture and heat for 4–5 minutes, or until the egg whites are scrambled and cooked through.
5. After turning off the heat, move the scramble to a platter.
6. Enjoy and warm up!

Recipe 3:

Egg White Scramble with Tomato and Spinach Veggie

Per-serving Nutritional Information:
- 150 calories

- 5g of total fat
- 1g of saturated fat
- There is no cholesterol.
- 330 mg of sodium
- 10g of carbohydrates
- 3g of fiber
- 6g of sugars
17g of protein

15 minutes for cooking
Serving Dimensions: 1

Components:
- One teaspoon of extra virgin olive oil
- Half a cup of cherry tomatoes
- One cup of raw spinach
- Egg whites, 3/4 cup (about 6 big egg whites)
To taste, add salt and pepper.

Guidelines:
1. In a nonstick skillet, warm the olive oil over medium heat.
2. When the cherry tomatoes begin to soften, add them to the skillet and simmer for two to three minutes.
3. Cook the fresh spinach leaves in the skillet for a further one to two minutes, or until they have wilted.
4. Add salt and pepper to taste and pour the egg whites into the skillet.
5. Gently stir the mixture and heat for 3–4 minutes, or until the egg whites are scrambled and cooked through.
6. After turning off the heat, move the scramble to a platter.
7. Enjoy and warm up!

Recipe 4:

Vegetable Egg White Scramble with Broccoli and Mushrooms

Per-serving Nutritional Information:
- 170 calories
- 6g of total fat
- 1g of saturated fat
- There is no cholesterol.
- 320 mg of sodium
- 11g of carbohydrates
- 4g of fiber
- 4g of sugars
19g of protein

20 minutes for cooking
Serving Dimensions: 1

Components:
- One teaspoon of extra virgin olive oil
- 1/2 cup of florets of broccoli
- 1/4 cup of mushroom slices
- Egg whites, 3/4 cup (about 6 big egg whites)
To taste, add salt and pepper.

Guidelines:
1. In a nonstick skillet, warm the olive oil over medium heat.
2. Place the sliced mushrooms and broccoli florets in the skillet and cook for 4–5 minutes, or until they are soft.
3. Add salt and pepper to taste and pour the egg whites into the skillet.
4. Gently stir the mixture and heat for 4–5 minutes, or until the egg whites are scrambled and cooked through.
5. After turning off the heat, move the scramble to a platter.
6. Enjoy and warm up!

Chia Seed Pudding with Berries

Recipe 1:

Chia Seed Pudding with Mixed Berries

Per-serving Nutritional Information:
- 220 calories
- 10g of total fat
- 1g of saturated fat
- There is no cholesterol.
- 40 milligrams of sodium
- 26g of carbohydrates
- 12g of fiber
- 10g of sugars
Six grams of protein

Overnight Cooking (with a 10-minute prep)
Serving Dimensions: 1

Components:
One-fourth cup chia seeds
- One cup of almond milk, without sugar added (or any other milk of your choosing)
- One tablespoon of optionally sweet maple syrup
- Half a teaspoon of essence from vanilla
- A half cup of mixed berries, including raspberries, blueberries, and strawberries

Guidelines:
1. The chia seeds, almond milk, vanilla extract, and maple syrup (if used) should all be combined in a bowl. Mix thoroughly to blend.
2. To keep the chia seeds from clumping, let the mixture sit for five minutes before stirring it once more.

3. Chia seeds swell and take on the consistency of pudding when they are covered and chilled for at least 4–6 hours or overnight.
4. Make sure to thoroughly mix the chia seed mixture before serving in order to break up any possible clumps.
5. Arrange the mixed berries and chia seed pudding in a serving bowl or glass.
6. Enjoy and serve cold!

Recipe 2:

Chia Seed Pudding with Strawberries

Per-serving Nutritional Information:
- 240 calories
- 11g of total fat
- 1g of saturated fat
- There is no cholesterol.
- 40 milligrams of sodium
- 30g of carbohydrates
- 12g of fiber
- 12g of sugars
Six grams of protein

Overnight Cooking (with a 10-minute prep)
Serving Dimensions: 1

Components:
One-fourth cup chia seeds
- One cup of almond milk, without sugar added (or any other milk of your choosing)
- One tablespoon of honey or your preferred sweetener
- Half a teaspoon of essence from vanilla
- Half a cup of freshly cut strawberries

Guidelines:

1. The chia seeds, almond milk, vanilla extract, honey, or other sweetener should all be combined in a bowl. Mix thoroughly to blend.
2. To keep the chia seeds from clumping, let the mixture sit for five minutes before stirring it once more.
3. Chia seeds swell and take on the consistency of pudding when they are covered and chilled for at least 4–6 hours or overnight.
4. Make sure to thoroughly mix the chia seed mixture before serving in order to break up any possible clumps.
5. Arrange the sliced strawberries and chia seed pudding in a serving bowl or glass.
6. Enjoy and serve cold!

Recipe 3:

Chia Seed Pudding with Blueberries

Per-serving Nutritional Information:
- 230 calories
- 11g of total fat
- 1g of saturated fat
- There is no cholesterol.
- 40 milligrams of sodium
- 29g of carbohydrates
- 12g of fiber
11g of sugars
Six grams of protein

Overnight Cooking (with a 10-minute prep)
Serving Dimensions: 1

Components:
One-fourth cup chia seeds
- One cup of almond milk, without sugar added (or any other milk of your choosing)
- One tablespoon of your preferred sweetener or agave syrup

- Half a teaspoon of essence from vanilla
- One-half cup of raw blueberries

Guidelines:
1. Chia seeds, almond milk, vanilla extract, and agave syrup (or other sweetener) should all be combined in a bowl. Mix thoroughly to blend.
2. To keep the chia seeds from clumping, let the mixture sit for five minutes before stirring it once more.
3. Chia seeds swell and take on the consistency of pudding when they are covered and chilled for at least 4–6 hours or overnight.
4. Make sure to thoroughly mix the chia seed mixture before serving in order to break up any possible clumps.
5. Arrange the fresh blueberries and chia seed pudding in a serving bowl or glass.
6. Enjoy and serve cold!

Whole Grain Avocado Toast:

Recipe 1:

Traditional Avocado Toast

Per-serving Nutritional Information:
- 250 calories
- 15g of total fat
- 2g of saturated fat
- There is no cholesterol.
- 200 milligrams of sodium
- 25g of carbohydrates
- 9g of fiber
- 2g of sugars
- 7g of protein

Five minutes for cooking

Serving Dimensions: 1

Components:
One piece of bread with healthy grains
- One mature avocado
- Juiced half a lemon
To taste, add salt and pepper.
- Adding sliced tomatoes, red pepper flakes, or sprouts is optional.

Guidelines:
1. Toast the whole grain bread until it reaches the crispiness you like.
2. Cut up the ripe avocado and remove the pit while the bread is browning. Remove the meat and place it in a basin.
3. Using a fork, mash the avocado until the appropriate consistency is achieved.
4. Add the half-lemon juice to the mashed avocado and stir thoroughly.
5. To taste, add salt and pepper to the avocado mixture.
6. After toasting the bread, evenly distribute the mashed avocado over it.
7. Top with optional ingredients like sprouts, red pepper flakes, or sliced tomatoes.
8. Enjoy and serve right now!

Recipe 2:

Avocado Toast with Mediterranean Flavors

Per-serving Nutritional Information:
- 320 calories
- 19g of total fat
- 3g of saturated fat
- There is no cholesterol.
- 360 mg of sodium
- 30g of carbohydrates
- 10g of fiber
- 3g of sugars

- 10g of protein

Ten minutes for cooking
Serving Dimensions: 1

Components:
One piece of bread with healthy grains
- One mature avocado
- Juiced half a lemon
To taste, add salt and pepper.
- Two tablespoons of feta cheese, crumbled
TWO TTS chopped Kalamata olives
- Two tablespoons of finely chopped sun-dried tomato
– New basil leaves as a finishing touch

Guidelines:
1. Toast the whole grain bread until it reaches the crispiness you like.
2. Cut up the ripe avocado and remove the pit while the bread is browning. Remove the meat and place it in a basin.
3. Using a fork, mash the avocado until the appropriate consistency is achieved.
4. Add the half-lemon juice to the mashed avocado and stir thoroughly.
5. To taste, add salt and pepper to the avocado mixture.
6. After toasting the bread, evenly distribute the mashed avocado over it.
7. Over the avocado, scatter chopped sun-dried tomatoes, chopped Kalamata olives, and crumbled feta cheese.
8. Add some fresh basil leaves as garnish.
9. Enjoy and serve right now!

Recipe 3:

Toast with spicy avocado

Per-serving Nutritional Information:
- 280 calories

- 16g of total fat
- 3g of saturated fat
- There is no cholesterol.
- 350 mg of sodium
- 31g of carbohydrates
- 11g of fiber
- 3g of sugars
- 8g of protein

Ten minutes for cooking
Serving Dimensions: 1

Components:
One piece of bread with healthy grains
- One mature avocado
- Juiced half a lemon
To taste, add salt and pepper.
- Half a teaspoon of chile powder
- One tablespoon of freshly chopped cilantro
- One tablespoon of finely chopped queso fresco (or any other preferred cheese)

Guidelines:
1. Toast the whole grain bread until it reaches the crispiness you like.
2. Cut up the ripe avocado and remove the pit while the bread is browning. Remove the meat and place it in a basin.
3. Using a fork, mash the avocado until the appropriate consistency is achieved.
4. Add the half-lemon juice to the mashed avocado and stir thoroughly.
5. To taste, add salt and pepper to the avocado mixture.
6. After toasting the bread, evenly distribute the mashed avocado over it.
7. Over the avocado, scatter chopped fresh cilantro and chili flakes.
8. Top with a crumble of queso fresco or your preferred cheese.
9. Enjoy and serve right now!

CHAPTER TWO

Healthy Lunches

Salad with quinoa and roasted vegetables:

Recipe 1:

Traditional Quinoa Salad with Roasted Vegetables

Per-serving Nutritional Information:
- 350 calories
- 12g of total fat
- 2g of saturated fat
- There is no cholesterol.
- 400 mg of sodium
- 50g of carbohydrates
- 9g of fiber
- 8g of sugars
12g of protein

40 minutes for cooking
Serving Dimensions: 1

Components:
- A cup of prepared quinoa

- One cup of mixed roasted veggies, including red onions, bell peppers, zucchini, and eggplant
- 1/4 cup of feta cheese, crumbled
- Two teaspoons of finely chopped fresh herbs, like basil or parsley
- Two teaspoons pure olive oil
- One tablespoon of juiced lemon
To taste, add salt and pepper.

Guidelines:
1. Set oven temperature to 400°F, or 200°C.
2. After spreading some olive oil over the mixed vegetables on a baking sheet, season with salt and pepper. For an even coat, toss.
3. For about 25 to 30 minutes, or until they are soft and beginning to caramelize, roast the vegetables in a preheated oven.
4. Mix the cooked quinoa, feta cheese crumbles, chopped fresh herbs, and roasted veggies in a big bowl.
5. To make the dressing, combine the olive oil, lemon juice, salt, and pepper in a small bowl.
6. Toss carefully to ensure that everything is uniformly coated after adding the dressing to the quinoa and vegetable mixture.
7. If necessary, adjust the seasoning.
8. To let the flavors mingle together, serve the salad right away or chill it for a few hours.
9. Have fun!

Recipe 2:

Roasted Vegetable Salad with Quinoa and Mediterranean Flavors

Per-serving Nutritional Information:
- 320 calories
- 10g of total fat
- 2g of saturated fat
- There is no cholesterol.
- 350 mg of sodium

- 48g of carbohydrates
- 9g of fiber
- 10g of sugars
- 11g of protein

45 minutes for cooking
Serving Dimensions: 1

Components:
- A cup of prepared quinoa
- One cup of mixed roasted veggies, including kalamata olives, cucumbers, red onions, and cherry tomatoes
- 1/4 cup of feta cheese, crumbled
- Two tablespoons of freshly chopped parsley
- Two tablespoons of freshly chopped mint
- Two teaspoons pure olive oil
- One tablespoon of juiced lemon
To taste, add salt and pepper.

Guidelines:
1. Set oven temperature to 400°F, or 200°C.
2. Arrange the red onion, cucumber, and cherry tomatoes on a baking sheet; toss to coat, then sprinkle with salt and pepper. For an even coat, toss.
3. For about 15 to 20 minutes, or until the other veggies are soft and the tomatoes have developed a tiny blister, roast the vegetables in the preheated oven.
4. The cooked quinoa, roasted veggies, crumbled feta cheese, chopped fresh parsley, and chopped fresh mint should all be combined in a big bowl.
5. To make the dressing, combine the olive oil, lemon juice, salt, and pepper in a small bowl.
6. Toss carefully to ensure that everything is uniformly coated after adding the dressing to the quinoa and vegetable mixture.
7. If necessary, adjust the seasoning.

8. To let the flavors mingle together, serve the salad right away or chill it for a few hours.
9. Have fun!

Recipe 3:

Quinoa and Roasted Vegetable Salad with Asian Infusion

Per-serving Nutritional Information:
- 330 calories
- 11g of total fat
- 2g of saturated fat
- There is no cholesterol.
- 450 mg of sodium
- 49g of carbohydrates
- 9g of fiber
- 12g of sugars
- 10g of protein

40 minutes for cooking
Serving Dimensions: 1

Components:
- A cup of prepared quinoa
- One cup of mixed roasted veggies, including carrots, bell peppers, broccoli, and snow peas
- Two teaspoons of thinly sliced onion
- Two tablespoons of freshly cut cilantro
- Two tablespoons of sesame oil, toasted
- A tablespoon of soy sauce with reduced sodium
- One tablespoon vinegar made with rice
- One tsp honey
To taste, add salt and pepper.
1 A garnish of sesame seeds

Guidelines:

1. Set oven temperature to 400°F, or 200°C.

2. After spreading some olive oil over the mixed vegetables on a baking sheet, season with salt and pepper. For an even coat, toss.

3. Bake the vegetables for 20 to 25 minutes, or until they are soft and beginning to take on some color, in a preheated oven.

4. The cooked quinoa, roasted veggies, sliced green onions, and freshly cut cilantro should all be combined in a big bowl.

5. To prepare the dressing, combine the soy sauce, honey, rice vinegar, toasted sesame oil, salt, and pepper in a small bowl.

6. Toss carefully to ensure that everything is uniformly coated after adding the dressing to the quinoa and vegetable mixture.

7. If necessary, adjust the seasoning.

8. As a garnish, add a little sesame seed sprinkle.

9. To let the flavors mingle together, serve the salad right away or chill it for a few hours.

10. Have fun!

Recipe 4:

Roasted Vegetable Salad with Southwest Quinoa

Per-serving Nutritional Information:
- 380 calories
- 15g of total fat
- 2g of saturated fat
- There is no cholesterol.
- 520 mg of sodium
- 50g of carbohydrates
- 10g of fiber
- 9g of sugars
12g of protein

45 minutes for cooking
Serving Dimensions: 1

Components:
- A cup of prepared quinoa
- One cup of mixed roasted veggies, including black beans, corn, bell peppers, and red onions
- 1/4 cup of avocado, diced
- Two tablespoons of freshly cut cilantro
- Two teaspoons of juiced lime
- One tablespoon pure olive oil
- One tsp of chili powder
- Half a teaspoon of cumin
To taste, add salt and pepper.
- Additions: shredded cheese, sour cream, and chopped jalapeños

Guidelines:
1. Set oven temperature to 400°F, or 200°C.
2. Spread a baking sheet with the mixed vegetables, cover with olive oil, and season with cumin, chili powder, salt, and pepper. For an even coat, toss.
3. Bake the vegetables for 20 to 25 minutes, or until they are soft and beginning to take on some color, in a preheated oven.
4. The cooked quinoa, diced avocado, chopped fresh cilantro, and roasted veggies should all be combined in a big bowl.
5. To prepare the dressing, combine the lime juice, olive oil, salt, and pepper in a small bowl.
6. Toss carefully to ensure that everything is uniformly coated after adding the dressing to the quinoa and vegetable mixture.
7. If necessary, adjust the seasoning.
8. To let the flavors mingle together, serve the salad right away or chill it for a few hours.
9. Adding sliced jalapeños, sour cream, or shredded cheese on top is optional but adds flavor and texture.
10. Have fun!

Grilled Chicken Wraps with Lemon Herbs:

Recipe 1:

Traditional Grilled Chicken Wrap with Lemon Herbs

Per-serving Nutritional Information:
- 350 calories
- 10g of total fat
- 2g of saturated fat
- 65 mg of cholesterol
- 700 mg of sodium
- 35g of carbohydrates
- 4g of fiber
- 5g of sugars
- 30g of protein

25 minutes for cooking
Serving Size: One Wrap

Components:
- Four ounces of sliced, grilled chicken breast
One whole-wheat tortilla
- Two tsp Greek yogurt
A tsp of freshly squeezed lemon juice
- One tsp lemon zest
- One teaspoon of freshly chopped dill
- One teaspoon of freshly chopped parsley
To taste, add salt and pepper.
1/4 cup of chopped lettuce
- Two tomato slices
- Two red onion slices

Guidelines:

1. To make the lemon herb sauce, combine the Greek yogurt, lemon juice, lemon zest, dill, parsley, salt, and pepper in a small bowl.
2. Spread out the whole wheat tortilla.
3. Evenly distribute the lemon-herb sauce onto the tortilla.
4. Arrange the slices of grilled chicken over the sauce.
5. Place the tomato slices, red onion slices, and shredded lettuce on top of the chicken.
6. Tuck the sides in as you carefully roll up the tortilla.
7. Cut the wrapper in half on the diagonal.
8. Serve right away or cover with foil to eat later.
9. Have fun!

Recipe 2:

Grilled Chicken Wrap with Greek Lemon Herbs

Per-serving Nutritional Information:
- 380 calories
- 12g of total fat
- 3g of saturated fat
- 65 mg of cholesterol
- 800 mg of sodium
- 40g of carbohydrates
- 5g of fiber
- 6g of sugars
- 30g of protein

25 minutes for cooking
Serving Size: One Wrap

Components:
- Four ounces of sliced, grilled chicken breast
One whole-wheat tortilla
- Two tablespoons of sauce (tzatziki)
A tsp of freshly squeezed lemon juice

- One tsp lemon zest
- One teaspoon of freshly chopped dill
To taste, add salt and pepper.
- 1/4 cup of cucumber, diced
1/4 cup of tomatoes, diced
- Two tablespoons of feta cheese, crumbled
- Two tablespoons of Kalamata olives, sliced
- Two tablespoons of freshly chopped parsley

Guidelines:
1. To make the lemon herb sauce, combine the tzatziki sauce, lemon juice, lemon zest, dill, salt, and pepper in a small bowl.
2. Spread out the whole wheat tortilla.
3. Over the tortilla, equally distribute the tzatziki sauce.
4. Arrange the slices of grilled chicken over the sauce.
5. Over the chicken, scatter the chopped fresh parsley, diced cucumber, diced tomatoes, crumbled feta cheese, and sliced Kalamata olives.
6. Tuck the sides in as you carefully roll up the tortilla.
7. Cut the wrapper in half on the diagonal.
8. Serve right away or cover with foil to eat later.
9. Have fun!

Recipe 3:

Grilled Chicken Wrap with Caesar Salad and Herbs

Per-serving Nutritional Information:
- 370 calories
- 13g of total fat
- 3g of saturated fat
- 65 mg of cholesterol
- 800 mg of sodium
- 35g of carbohydrates
- 4g of fiber
- 3g of sugars

- 30g of protein

25 minutes for cooking
Serving Size: One Wrap

Components:
- Four ounces of sliced, grilled chicken breast
One whole-wheat tortilla
- Two teaspoons of Caesar salad
A tsp of freshly squeezed lemon juice
- One tsp lemon zest
- One teaspoon of freshly chopped parsley
To taste, add salt and pepper.
- 1/4 cup of romaine lettuce, shredded
- Two tsp finely grated Parmesan cheese
- Twice as many croutons

Guidelines:
1. To make the lemon herb sauce, combine the Caesar dressing, lemon juice, lemon zest, parsley, salt, and pepper in a small bowl.
2. Spread out the whole wheat tortilla.
3. Evenly distribute the Caesar dressing sauce onto the tortilla.
4. Arrange the slices of grilled chicken over the sauce.
5. Over the chicken, scatter the croutons, grated Parmesan cheese, and shredded romaine lettuce.
6. Tuck the sides in as you carefully roll up the tortilla.
7. Cut the wrapper in half on the diagonal.
8. Serve right away or store in foil for later.
9. Have fun!

Recipe 4:

Grilled Chicken Wrap with Spicy Lemon Herbs

Per-serving Nutritional Information:

- 360 calories
- 11g of total fat
- 2g of saturated fat
- 65 mg of cholesterol
- 900 mg of sodium
- 38g of carbohydrates
- 5g of fiber
- 4g of sugars
- 30g of protein

25 minutes for cooking
Serving Size: One Wrap

Components:
- Four ounces of sliced, grilled chicken breast
One whole-wheat tortilla
- Two teaspoons hot mayonnaise
A tsp of freshly squeezed lemon juice
- One tsp lemon zest
- One teaspoon of freshly chopped cilantro
- One-half teaspoon of chili powder
To taste, add salt and pepper.
- 1/4 cup of bell peppers, thinly sliced
- 1/4 cup of red onion, thinly sliced
- Two teaspoons of jalapeños, sliced
- Two tablespoons of freshly chopped parsley

Guidelines:
1. To make the lemon herb sauce, combine the spicy mayo, lemon juice, zest, cilantro, chili powder, salt, and pepper in a small bowl.
2. Spread out the whole wheat tortilla.
3. Over the tortilla, equally distribute the hot mayonnaise sauce.
4. Arrange the slices of grilled chicken over the sauce.
5. Over the chicken, scatter the sliced bell peppers, red onion, sliced jalapeños, and chopped fresh parsley.

6. Tuck the sides in as you carefully roll up the tortilla.
7. Cut the wrapper in half on the diagonal.
8. Serve right away or cover with foil to eat later.
9. Have fun!

Mediterranean Salad with Chickpeas:

Recipe 1:

Inventive Mediterranean Chickpea Salad

Per-serving Nutritional Information:
- 250 calories
- 10g of total fat
- 1g of saturated fat
- There is no cholesterol.
- 450 mg of sodium
- 32g of carbohydrates
- 8g of fiber
- 6g of sugars
- 9g of protein

15 minutes for cooking
One cup is the serving size.

Components:
One can (15 ounces) of rinsed and drained chickpeas
One cup of cucumbers, diced
Diced tomatoes, one cup
- 1/2 cup of red onion, chopped
- One-half cup of chopped bell pepper, any color
- 1/4 cup of halved and pitted Kalamata olives
- 1/4 cup of feta cheese, crumbled
- Two tablespoons of freshly chopped parsley

– Two tsp extra virgin olive oil
A tsp of freshly squeezed lemon juice
- One minced garlic clove
- Half a teaspoon of oregano, dry
To taste, add salt and pepper.

Guidelines:
1. Chickpeas, cucumber, tomatoes, bell pepper, red onion, Kalamata olives, feta cheese, and parsley should all be combined in a big bowl.
2. Mix the olive oil, lemon juice, dried oregano, minced garlic, salt, and pepper in a small bowl.
3. After adding the dressing to the chickpea mixture, gently toss to mix.
4. If necessary, adjust the seasoning.
5. To allow the flavors to mingle, let the salad sit for a minimum of ten minutes.
6. Serve either room temperature or cold.
7. Have fun!

Recipe 2:

Greek Mediterranean Chickpea Salad

Per-serving Nutritional Information:
- 280 calories
- 12g of total fat
- 2g of saturated fat
- There is no cholesterol.
- 500 milligrams of sodium
- 35g of carbohydrates
- 9g of fiber
- 6g of sugars
- 11g of protein

15 minutes for cooking
One cup is the serving size.

Components:
One can (15 ounces) of rinsed and drained chickpeas
One cup of cucumbers, diced
Diced tomatoes, one cup
- 1/2 cup of red onion, chopped
- One-half cup of chopped bell pepper, any color
- 1/4 cup of halved and pitted Kalamata olives
- 1/4 cup of feta cheese, crumbled
- Two tablespoons of freshly chopped parsley
– Two tsp extra virgin olive oil
A tsp of freshly squeezed lemon juice
- One minced garlic clove
- One teaspoon of oregano, dried
To taste, add salt and pepper.

Guidelines:
1. Chickpeas, cucumber, tomatoes, bell pepper, red onion, Kalamata olives, feta cheese, and parsley should all be combined in a big bowl.
2. Mix the olive oil, lemon juice, dried oregano, minced garlic, salt, and pepper in a small bowl.
3. After adding the dressing to the chickpea mixture, gently toss to mix.
4. If necessary, adjust the seasoning.
5. To allow the flavors to mingle, let the salad sit for a minimum of ten minutes.
6. Serve either room temperature or cold.
7. Have fun!

Recipe 3:

Mediterranean Chickpea Salad with Avocado

Per-serving Nutritional Information:
- 320 calories
- 16g of total fat

- 2g of saturated fat
- There is no cholesterol.
- 450 mg of sodium
- 35g of carbohydrates
- 10g of fiber
- 6g of sugars
- 9g of protein

15 minutes for cooking
One cup is the serving size.

Components:
One can (15 ounces) of rinsed and drained chickpeas
One cup of cucumbers, diced
Diced tomatoes, one cup
- 1/2 cup of red onion, chopped
- One-half cup of chopped bell pepper, any color
- 1/4 cup of halved and pitted Kalamata olives
- 1/4 cup of feta cheese, crumbled
- Two tablespoons of freshly chopped parsley
– Two tsp extra virgin olive oil
A tsp of freshly squeezed lemon juice
- One minced garlic clove
- One sliced ripe avocado
To taste, add salt and pepper.

Guidelines:
1. Chickpeas, cucumber, tomatoes, bell pepper, red onion, Kalamata olives, feta cheese, and parsley should all be combined in a big bowl.
2. Mix the olive oil, lemon juice, minced garlic, salt, and pepper in a small bowl.
3. After adding the dressing to the chickpea mixture, gently toss to mix.
4. Fold in the cubed avocado gently.
5. If necessary, adjust the seasoning.

6. To allow the flavors to mingle, let the salad sit for a minimum of ten minutes.
7. Serve either room temperature or cold.
8. Have fun!

Recipe 4:

Quinoa Chickpea Salad with Mediterranean Flavors

Per-serving Nutritional Information:
- 320 calories
- 12g of total fat
- 2g of saturated fat
- There is no cholesterol.
- 400 mg of sodium
- 45g of carbohydrates
- 10g of fiber
- 6g of sugars
- 11g of protein

25 minutes for cooking
One cup is the serving size.

Components:
- A cup of prepared quinoa
One can (15 ounces) of rinsed and drained chickpeas
One cup of cucumbers, diced
Diced tomatoes, one cup
- 1/2 cup of red onion, chopped
- One-half cup of chopped bell pepper, any color
- 1/4 cup of halved and pitted Kalamata olives
- 1/4 cup of feta cheese, crumbled
- Two tablespoons of freshly chopped parsley
– Two tsp extra virgin olive oil

To taste, add salt and pepper.

Guidelines:
1. The cooked quinoa, chickpeas, cucumber, tomatoes, bell pepper, red onion, Kalamata olives, feta cheese, and parsley should all be combined in a big bowl.
2. Mix the olive oil, lemon juice, dried oregano, minced garlic, salt, and pepper in a small bowl.
3. After adding the dressing to the quinoa and chickpea mixture, gently toss to blend.
4. If necessary, adjust the seasoning.
5. To allow the flavors to mingle, let the salad sit for a minimum of ten minutes.
6. Serve either room temperature or cold.
7. Have fun!

Salmon on the grill with dill yogurt sauce:

Recipe 1:

Traditional Dill Yogurt Sauce Grilled Salmon

Per-serving Nutritional Information:
- 350 calories
- 20g of total fat
- 4g of saturated fat
- 90 mg of cholesterol
- 400 mg of sodium
- 5g of carbohydrates
- Fiber: 0 g
- 3g of sugars
35g of protein

15 minutes for cooking

One fillet served at a time

Components:
- Four six-ounce salmon fillets each
To taste, add salt and pepper.
- One tablespoon of olive oil

Regarding the Yogurt Dill Sauce:
- One cup of Greek yogurt, plain
- Two tablespoons of freshly chopped dill
A tsp of freshly squeezed lemon juice
- One minced garlic clove
To taste, add salt and pepper.

Guidelines:
1. Set the grill's temperature to medium-high.
2. Olive oil, salt, and pepper are used to season the salmon fillets.
3. The salmon fillets should be cooked through and flake readily with a fork after about 4–5 minutes of cooking on each side on a hot grill.
4. Make the dill yogurt sauce while the salmon is grilling.
5. Greek yogurt, minced garlic, lemon juice, chopped dill, salt, and pepper should all be combined in a small basin. Blend thoroughly.
6. After the salmon is done, take it off the grill and give it some time to rest.
7. Arrange the grilled fish onto a plate and drizzle with dill yogurt sauce.
8. Have fun!

Recipe 2:

Grilled Salmon with Lemon Herbs and Dill Yogurt Sauce

Per-serving Nutritional Information:
- 380 calories
- 22g of total fat
- 4g of saturated fat
- 90 mg of cholesterol

- 400 mg of sodium
- 5g of carbohydrates
- Fiber: 0 g
- 3g of sugars
38g of protein

15 minutes for cooking
One fillet served at a time

Components:
- Four six-ounce salmon fillets each
To taste, add salt and pepper.
- One tablespoon of olive oil
- One lemon's zest
- Two teaspoons of finely chopped fresh herbs (parsley, basil, or thyme)

Regarding the Yogurt Dill Sauce:
- One cup of Greek yogurt, plain
- Two tablespoons of freshly chopped dill
A tsp of freshly squeezed lemon juice
- One minced garlic clove
To taste, add salt and pepper.

Guidelines:
1. Set the grill's temperature to medium-high.
2. Salt, pepper, olive oil, lemon zest, and finely chopped fresh herbs are used to season the salmon fillets.
3. The salmon fillets should be cooked through and flake readily with a fork after about 4–5 minutes of cooking on each side on a hot grill.
4. Make the dill yogurt sauce while the salmon is grilling.
5. Greek yogurt, minced garlic, lemon juice, chopped dill, salt, and pepper should all be combined in a small basin. Blend thoroughly.
6. After the salmon is done, take it off the grill and give it some time to rest.
7. Arrange the grilled fish onto a plate and drizzle with dill yogurt sauce.
8. Have fun!

Recipe 3:

Dill Yogurt Sauce and Spicy Cajun Grilled Salmon

Per-serving Nutritional Information:
- 380 calories
- 22g of total fat
- 4g of saturated fat
- 90 mg of cholesterol
- 400 mg of sodium
- 5g of carbohydrates
- Fiber: 0 g
- 3g of sugars
38g of protein

15 minutes for cooking
One fillet served at a time

Components:
- Four six-ounce salmon fillets each
To taste, add salt and pepper.
- One tablespoon of olive oil
- One tablespoon of Cajun spice

Regarding the Yogurt Dill Sauce:
- One cup of Greek yogurt, plain
- Two tablespoons of freshly chopped dill
A tsp of freshly squeezed lemon juice
- One minced garlic clove
To taste, add salt and pepper.

Guidelines:
1. Set the grill's temperature to medium-high.
2. Add salt, pepper, olive oil, and Cajun seasoning to the salmon fillets.

3. The salmon fillets should be cooked through and flake readily with a fork after about 4–5 minutes of cooking on each side on a hot grill.
4. Make the dill yogurt sauce while the salmon is grilling.
5. Greek yogurt, minced garlic, lemon juice, chopped dill, salt, and pepper should all be combined in a small basin. Blend thoroughly.
6. After the salmon is done, take it off the grill and give it some time to rest.
7. Arrange the grilled fish onto a plate and drizzle with dill yogurt sauce.
8. Have fun!

Recipe 4:

Dill Yogurt Sauce with Grilled Salmon Glazed with Maple

Per-serving Nutritional Information:
- 400 calories
- 22g of total fat
- 4g of saturated fat
- 90 mg of cholesterol
- 400 mg of sodium
- 10g of carbohydrates
- Fiber: 0 g
- 9g of sugars
35g of protein

15 minutes for cooking
One fillet served at a time

Components:
- Four six-ounce salmon fillets each
To taste, add salt and pepper.
- Two tsp pure maple syrup
Soy sauce (one tablespoon)
- One tablespoon of mustard dijon

Regarding the Yogurt Dill Sauce:

- One cup of Greek yogurt, plain
- Two tablespoons of freshly chopped dill
A tsp of freshly squeezed lemon juice
- One minced garlic clove
To taste, add salt and pepper.

Guidelines:
1. Set the grill's temperature to medium-high.
2. Use salt and pepper to season the salmon fillets.
3. Mix the soy sauce, Dijon mustard, and maple syrup in a small basin.
4. To ensure equal coating, brush the salmon fillets with the maple glaze mixture.
5. The salmon fillets should be cooked through and flake readily with a fork after about 4–5 minutes of cooking on each side on a hot grill.
6. Make the dill yogurt sauce while the salmon is grilling.
7. Greek yogurt, minced garlic, lemon juice, chopped dill, salt, and pepper should all be combined in a small basin. Blend thoroughly.
8. After the salmon is done, take it off the grill and give it some time to rest.
9. Arrange the grilled fish onto a plate and drizzle with dill yogurt sauce.
10. Have fun!

CHAPTER THREE

Filling Meals

Herbed Quinoa with Baked Cod

Recipe 1:

Herbed Quinoa with Baked Cod

Information about Nutrition:
- 300 calories each serving
25g of protein
- 30g of carbohydrates
- 8g of fat
- 30 minutes for cooking
- Portion Size: Four portions

Components:
– 4 fish fillets, each weighing 4-6 ounces
- One cup of washed quinoa
- Two cups broth made of vegetables
- Two teaspoons of finely chopped fresh herbs (such basil, dill, or parsley)
- One divided lemon
- Two tsp olive oil
To taste, add salt and pepper.

Guidelines:
1. Turn the oven on to 375°F, or 190°C.
2. Add salt, pepper, and the juice from half a lemon to the cod fillets. Put aside.

3. The vegetable broth should be brought to a boil in a saucepan. When the quinoa is cooked and the liquid has been absorbed, add it, lower the heat to low, cover it, and simmer for 15 to 20 minutes.

4. Add the chopped fresh herbs, half a lemon's zest, and a tablespoon of olive oil to a small bowl. Blend thoroughly.

5. Arrange the seasoned cod fillets on an aluminum foil or parchment paper-lined baking sheet.

6. Garnish each cod fillet with a little of the herb mixture.

7. Bake the fish for 12 to 15 minutes in a preheated oven, or until it is cooked through and flake easily with a fork.

8. In another bowl, toss the cooked quinoa with the juice from half a lemon, 1 tablespoon olive oil, salt, and pepper while the fish bakes. Blend thoroughly.

9. Arrange the roasted cod fillets onto a bed of quinoa with herbs.

10. If preferred, garnish with more fresh herbs.

11. Enjoy while hot!

Recipe 2:

Herbed Quinoa with Lemon-Garlic Baked Cod

Information about Nutrition:
- 280 calories each serving
28g of protein
- 30g of carbohydrates
- 7g of fat
- 30 minutes for cooking
- Portion Size: Four portions

Components:
– 4 fish fillets, each weighing 4-6 ounces
- One cup of washed quinoa
- Two cups broth made of vegetables
- Four minced garlic cloves
- Half a cup of lemon juice

- Two tsp olive oil
- One tablespoon of freshly chopped parsley
- One tsp lemon zest
To taste, add salt and pepper.

Guidelines:
1. Turn the oven on to 375°F, or 190°C.
2. Add minced garlic, salt, and pepper to the cod fillets' seasoning. Pour one tablespoon of olive oil and little lemon juice over it. Allow it to marinade for a short while.
3. The vegetable broth should be brought to a boil in a saucepan. When the quinoa is cooked and the liquid has been absorbed, add it, lower the heat to low, cover it, and simmer for 15 to 20 minutes.
4. Add the lemon zest, chopped parsley, salt, pepper, and a tablespoon of olive oil to a small bowl. Blend thoroughly.
5. Arrange the marinated cod fillets onto a baking sheet that has been covered with aluminum foil or parchment paper.
6. Garnish each cod fillet with a little of the herb mixture.
7. Bake the fish for 12 to 15 minutes in a preheated oven, or until it is cooked through and flake easily with a fork.
8. In a another bowl, mix the cooked quinoa with 1 tablespoon of lemon juice and salt to taste, while the cod bakes. Blend thoroughly.
9. On a bed of herbaceous quinoa, present the baked fish fillets with lemon and garlic.
10. If preferred, garnish with more parsley and lemon wedges.
11. Enjoy while hot!

Recipe 3:

Herbed Quinoa with Pesto-crusted Baked Cod

Information about Nutrition:
320 calories each serving
27g of protein
- 30g of carbohydrates

- 12g of fat
- 30 minutes for cooking
- Portion Size: Four portions

Components:
– 4 fish fillets, each weighing 4-6 ounces
- One cup of washed quinoa
- Two cups broth made of vegetables
– Four tsp pesto sauce
- Half a cup of lemon juice
- Two tsp olive oil
- One tablespoon of freshly chopped basil
To taste, add salt and pepper.

Guidelines:
1. Turn the oven on to 375°F, or 190°C.
2. Use lemon juice, salt, and pepper to season the cod fillets. Put aside.
3. The vegetable broth should be brought to a boil in a saucepan. Reduction of heat to low, cover, and simmer for 15 to 20 minutes is required after adding the quinoa. Recipe 4: Mediterranean Baked Cod with Herbed Quinoa

Information about Nutrition:
310 calories each serving
26g of protein
- 30g of carbohydrates
- 9g of fat
- 30 minutes for cooking
- Portion Size: Four portions

Components:
– 4 fish fillets, each weighing 4-6 ounces
- One cup of washed quinoa
- Two cups broth made of vegetables
- Two tsp olive oil

- Two minced garlic cloves
- One teaspoon of oregano, dried
- A teaspoon of thyme, dried
- One tsp of dried basil
One-half tsp paprika
To taste, add salt and pepper.
- One lemon's juice
- To garnish, fresh parsley

Guidelines:
1. Turn the oven on to 375°F, or 190°C.
2. Add minced garlic, salt, and pepper to the cod fillets' seasoning. Put aside.
3. The vegetable broth should be brought to a boil in a saucepan. When the quinoa is cooked and the liquid has been absorbed, add it, lower the heat to low, cover it, and simmer for 15 to 20 minutes.
4. Combine the olive oil, paprika, dried thyme, dried basil, dried oregano, dry pepper, and half a lemon's juice in a small bowl.
5. Arrange the seasoned cod fillets on an aluminum foil or parchment paper-lined baking sheet.
6. Drizzle each cod fillet with a mixture of olive oil and herbs.
7. Bake the fish for 12 to 15 minutes in a preheated oven, or until it is cooked through and flake easily with a fork.
8. In another bowl, toss the cooked quinoa with the juice from half a lemon, salt, and pepper while the fish bakes. Blend thoroughly.
9. Arrange the Mediterranean-style roasted cod fillets over a bed of quinoa with herbs.
10. Add fresh parsley as a garnish.
11. Enjoy while hot!

Bell Peppers Stuffed with Ratatouille

Recipe 1:

Stuffed bell peppers with Ratatouille

Information about Nutrition:
- 180 calories each serving
- 5g of protein
- 30g of carbohydrates
- 5g of fat
- 45 minutes for cooking
- Portion Size: Four portions

Components:
- Four bell peppers, any hue
- One little eggplant, chopped
- One diced zucchini
- One diced yellow squash
- One chopped onion
- Two minced garlic cloves
- One 14-oz can of chopped tomatoes
- One tablespoon of olive oil
- One tsp of dried basil
- One teaspoon of oregano, dried
To taste, add salt and pepper.
- Optional grated Parmesan cheese

Guidelines:
1. Turn the oven on to 375°F, or 190°C.
2. Slice off the bell peppers' tops, then take out the seeds and membranes.
3. Heat the olive oil in a big skillet over medium heat. Add the garlic and onion, and cook until aromatic and softened.

4. To the skillet, add the diced yellow squash, zucchini, and eggplant. Cook, stirring occasionally, until the vegetables begin to soften, about 5 minutes.
5. Add the diced tomatoes, salt, pepper, dried oregano, and dried basil. Mix thoroughly to blend.
6. Allow the mixture to gently cook for approximately ten minutes, or until the flavors have combined and the vegetables become soft.
7. Fill the prepared bell peppers to the brim with the ratatouille mixture using a spoon.
8. The filled peppers should be put in a baking dish and covered with foil.
9. Bake in the preheated oven for 30 minutes.
10. If desired, remove the foil and top each pepper with grated Parmesan cheese.
11. Bake the cheese for a further five minutes, or until it is melted and starting to turn golden.
12. Enjoy while hot!

Recipe 2:

Stuffed Bell Peppers with Quinoa

Information about Nutrition:
- Each serving has 220 calories.
- 9g of protein
- 38g of carbohydrates
- 5g of fat
- 50 minutes for cooking
- Portion Size: Four portions

Components:
- Four bell peppers, any hue
- One cup of washed quinoa
- Two cups broth made of vegetables
- One chopped onion
- Two minced garlic cloves
- One diced zucchini

- One grated carrot
Diced tomatoes, one cup
- One tsp of dried basil
- One teaspoon of oregano, dried
To taste, add salt and pepper.
- Optional grated cheese for topping

Guidelines:
1. Turn the oven on to 375°F, or 190°C.
2. Slice off the bell peppers' tops, then take out the seeds and membranes.
3. The vegetable broth should be brought to a boil in a saucepan. When the quinoa is cooked and the liquid has been absorbed, add it, lower the heat to low, cover it, and simmer for 15 to 20 minutes.
4. Heat some olive oil in a big skillet over medium heat. Add the garlic and onion, and cook until aromatic and softened.
5. To the skillet, add the chopped tomatoes, zucchini, carrot, dried oregano, dry basil, and salt and pepper. Cook, stirring occasionally, until the vegetables are soft, about 5 minutes.
6. The cooked quinoa and the veggie mixture should be combined in a large mixing bowl.
7. Fill the bell peppers to the brim with the quinoa mixture by spooning it in.
8. The filled peppers should be put in a roasting tray. Garnish each pepper with grated cheese, if you'd like.
9. Bake for 25 to 30 minutes in a preheated oven, or until the cheese is golden and melted and the peppers are soft.
10. Enjoy while hot!

Recipe 3:

Stuffed Bell Peppers with a Mediterranean Flavor

Information about Nutrition:
- 250 calories per serving.
12g of protein

- 30g of carbohydrates
- 10g of fat
- 50 minutes for cooking
- Portion Size: Four portions

Components:
- Four bell peppers, any hue
- A cup of prepared quinoa
- One cup washed and drained canned chickpeas
Diced tomatoes, one cup
- 1/2 cup of cucumbers, diced
- Chopped 1/4 cup of Kalamata olives
- 1/4 cup of feta cheese, crumbled
- Two tablespoons of freshly chopped parsley
- Half a cup of lemon juice
- Two tsp olive oil
- One teaspoon of oregano, dried
To taste, add salt and pepper.

Guidelines:
1. Turn the oven on to 375°F, or 190°C.
2. Slice off the bell peppers' tops, then take out the seeds and membranes.
3. Cooked quinoa, chickpeas, diced tomatoes, cucumber, feta cheese, Kalamata olives, parsley, lemon juice, olive oil, dried oregano, salt, and pepper should all be combined in a mixing bowl. Until all of the ingredients are combined evenly, thoroughly mix.
4. Fill the bell peppers all the way to the top with the quinoa mixture.
5. The filled peppers should be put on a baking tray and covered with foil.
6. Bake for thirty minutes in a preheated oven.
7. After removing the foil, bake the peppers for a further 10 to 15 minutes, or until they are soft and starting to brown.
8. Enjoy while hot!

Recipe 4:

Mexican Stuffed Bell Peppers

Information about Nutrition:
- 280 calories each serving
- 15g of protein
- 30g of carbohydrates
- 12g of fat
- 50 minutes for cooking
- Portion Size: Four portions

Components:
- Four bell peppers, any hue
- One cup of brown rice, cooked
- One cup of cooked, rinsed and drained black beans
- One cup of kernel corn
- 1/2 cup of tomatoes, diced
- 1/4 cup of red onion, chopped
- 1/4 cup of freshly chopped cilantro
- One tsp of chili powder
- Half a teaspoon of cumin powder
One-half tsp paprika
To taste, add salt and pepper.
- Shredded cheddar cheese (optional) for a topping
- Salsa and sour cream for serving (optional)

Guidelines:
1. Turn the oven on to 375°F, or 190°C.
2. Slice off the bell peppers' tops, then take out the seeds and membranes.
3. Cooked brown rice, black beans, corn kernels, diced tomatoes, red onion, cilantro, cumin, paprika, chili powder, and salt and pepper should all be combined in a mixing dish. Until all of the ingredients are combined evenly, thoroughly mix.
4. Fill the bell peppers to the brim with the rice and bean mixture.
5. The filled peppers should be put in a roasting tray. Garnish each pepper with shredded cheddar cheese, if you'd like.

6. Bake for thirty minutes in a preheated oven.

7. Take them out of the oven and give them some time to cool.

8. If preferred, serve hot with salsa and sour cream.

Tomato-Garlic Turkey Meatballs

Recipe 1:

Traditional Tomato-Basted Turkey Meatballs

Information about Nutrition:
- 250 calories per serving.
20g of protein
- 10g of carbohydrates
- 15g of fat
- 40 minutes for cooking
- Portion Size: Four portions

Components:
Regarding the Meatballs:
- One pound of turkey ground
- Half a cup of breadcrumbs
– 1/4 cup of Parmesan cheese, grated
- 1/4 cup of freshly chopped parsley
- 1/4 cup finely sliced onion
- One minced clove of garlic
- One lightly beaten egg
- Half a teaspoon of oregano, dry
To taste, add salt and pepper.

Regarding the Tomato Sauce:
- Two tsp olive oil
- One little onion, diced finely
- Two minced garlic cloves
- One 14-ounce can of crushed tomatoes

- One tsp of dried basil
- One teaspoon of oregano, dried
To taste, add salt and pepper.

Guidelines:
1. Turn the oven on to 375°F, or 190°C.
2. All of the meatball ingredients—ground turkey, breadcrumbs, Parmesan cheese, minced garlic, chopped onion, chopped parsley, egg, dried oregano, salt, and pepper—should be combined in a big dish. Until all of the ingredients are combined equally, thoroughly mix.
3. After forming the mixture into meatballs with a diameter of 1-2 inches, transfer them to a baking sheet covered with parchment paper.
4. The meatballs should be cooked through and lightly browned after 20 to 25 minutes of baking in a preheated oven.
5. Make the tomato sauce while the meatballs are baking. Heat the olive oil in a medium-sized saucepan over medium heat. Add the minced garlic and diced onion, and sauté until aromatic and softened.
6. To the pot, add the smashed tomatoes, salt, pepper, dried oregano, and dried basil. Mix thoroughly to blend.
7. To let the flavors melt together, lower the heat to low, cover the saucepan, and simmer for 15 to 20 minutes.
8. After cooking, add the meatballs to the tomato sauce and simmer for a further five minutes to let the flavors meld.
9. Serve the tomato-sauced turkey meatballs over cooked pasta or with crusty bread on the side.
10. If desired, garnish with extra finely chopped parsley.
11. Savor it hot!

Recipe 2:

Tomato Sauce-Basted Spicy Turkey Meatballs

Information about Nutrition:
- 280 calories each serving
22g of protein

- 12g of carbohydrates
- 16g of fat
- 40 minutes for cooking
- Portion Size: Four portions

Components:
Regarding the Meatballs:
- One pound of turkey ground
- Half a cup of breadcrumbs
– 1/4 cup of Parmesan cheese, grated
- 1/4 cup of freshly chopped cilantro
- 1/4 cup finely sliced onion
- One minced clove of garlic
- One lightly beaten egg
- One teaspoon ground cumin.
One-half tsp paprika
One-fourth teaspoon cayenne pepper, or to taste
To taste, add salt and pepper.

Regarding the Tomato Sauce:
- Two tsp olive oil
- One little onion, diced finely
- Two minced garlic cloves
- One 14-ounce can of crushed tomatoes
- One teaspoon of oregano, dried
- 1/2 teaspoon (or more, depending on taste) red pepper flakes
To taste, add salt and pepper.

Guidelines:
1. Turn the oven on to 375°F, or 190°C.
2. All of the meatball ingredients—ground turkey, breadcrumbs, Parmesan cheese, chopped onion, chopped cilantro, minced garlic, egg, paprika, cumin, cayenne, salt, and pepper—should be combined in a big bowl. Until all of the ingredients are combined equally, thoroughly mix.

3. After forming the mixture into meatballs with a diameter of 1-2 inches, transfer them to a baking sheet covered with parchment paper.

4. The meatballs should be cooked through and lightly browned after 20 to 25 minutes of baking in a preheated oven.

5. Make the tomato sauce while the meatballs are baking. Heat the olive oil in a medium-sized saucepan over medium heat. Add the minced garlic and diced onion, and sauté until aromatic and softened.

6. To the pot, add the smashed tomatoes, red pepper flakes, dry oregano, salt, and pepper. Mix thoroughly to blend.

7. To let the flavors melt together, lower the heat to low, cover the saucepan, and simmer for 15 to 20 minutes.

8. After cooking, add the meatballs to the tomato sauce and simmer for a further five minutes to let the flavors meld.

9. Serve the hot, tomato-sauced turkey meatballs with crusty bread on the side or over boiled rice.

10. If desired, garnish with extra finely chopped cilantro.

11. Savor it hot!

Recipe 3:

Tomato Sauced Italian Turkey Meatballs

Information about Nutrition:
- Each serving has 270 calories.
23g of protein
- 15g of carbohydrates
- 13g of fat
- 45 minutes for cooking
- Portion Size: Four portions

Components:
Regarding the Meatballs:
- One pound of turkey ground
- Half a cup of breadcrumbs
– 1/4 cup of Parmesan cheese, grated

- 1/4 cup of freshly chopped basil
- 1/4 cup finely sliced onion
- One minced clove of garlic
- One lightly beaten egg
- One teaspoon of oregano, dried
To taste, add salt and pepper.

Regarding the Tomato Sauce:
- Two tsp olive oil
- One little onion, diced finely
- Two minced garlic cloves
- One 14-ounce can of crushed tomatoes
- One tsp of dried basil
- One teaspoon of oregano, dried
To taste, add salt and pepper.

Guidelines:
1. Turn the oven on to 375°F, or 190°C.
2. All the components for the meatballs—ground turkey, breadcrumbs, Parmesan cheese, chopped onion, chopped basil, minced garlic, egg, dried oregano, salt, and pepper—should be combined in a big bowl. Until all of the ingredients are combined equally, thoroughly mix.
3. After forming the mixture into meatballs with a diameter of 1-2 inches, transfer them to a baking sheet covered with parchment paper.
4. The meatballs should be cooked through and lightly browned after 20 to 25 minutes of baking in a preheated oven.
5. Make the tomato sauce while the meatballs are baking. Heat the olive oil in a medium-sized saucepan over medium heat. Add the minced garlic and diced onion, and sauté until aromatic and softened.
6. To the pot, add the smashed tomatoes, salt, pepper, dried oregano, and dried basil. Mix thoroughly to blend.
7. To let the flavors melt together, lower the heat to low, cover the saucepan, and simmer for 15 to 20 minutes.
8. After cooking, add the meatballs to the tomato sauce and simmer for a further five minutes to let the flavors meld.

9. Serve the cooked spaghetti with the Italian-style turkey meatballs in tomato sauce on the side or over garlic bread.
10. If desired, garnish with more finely chopped basil.
11. Savor it hot!

Recipe 4:

Turkey Meatballs with Tomato Sauce and Greek Inspiration

Information about Nutrition:
- 290 calories each serving
24g of protein
- 14g of carbohydrates
- 15g of fat
- 40 minutes for cooking
- Portion Size: Four portions

Components:
Regarding the Meatballs:
- One pound of turkey ground
- Half a cup of breadcrumbs
- 1/4 cup of feta cheese, crumbled
- 1/4 cup of freshly chopped parsley
- 1/4 cup of red onion, chopped
- One minced clove of garlic
- One lightly beaten egg
- One teaspoon of oregano, dried
To taste, add salt and pepper.

Regarding the Tomato Sauce:
- Two tsp olive oil
- One little onion, diced finely
- Two minced garlic cloves
- One 14-ounce can of crushed tomatoes
- One teaspoon of oregano, dried

- One-half teaspoon of dried mint
To taste, add salt and pepper.

Guidelines:
1. Turn the oven on to 375°F, or 190°C.
2. All of the meatball ingredients—ground turkey, breadcrumbs, feta cheese, minced garlic, chopped red onion, chopped parsley, dried oregano, egg, salt, and pepper—should be combined in a big bowl. Until all of the ingredients are combined equally, thoroughly mix.
3. After forming the mixture into meatballs with a diameter of 1-2 inches, transfer them to a baking sheet covered with parchment paper.
4. The meatballs should be cooked through and lightly browned after 20 to 25 minutes of baking in a preheated oven.
5. Make the tomato sauce while the meatballs are baking. Heat the olive oil in a medium-sized saucepan over medium heat. Add the minced garlic and diced onion, and sauté until aromatic and softened.
6. To the pot, add the smashed tomatoes, salt, pepper, dried mint, and dried oregano. Mix thoroughly to blend.
7. To let the flavors melt together, lower the heat to low, cover the saucepan, and simmer for 15 to 20 minutes.

Goat cheese tart with roasted vegetables

Recipe 1:

Tart with roasted vegetables and goat cheese

Information about Nutrition:
- 300 calories each serving
- 10g of protein
- 30g of carbohydrates
- 16g of fat
– Prep Time: 60 minutes

- Quantity Per Serving: 6 pieces

Components:
One sheet of thawed puff pastry
- One cup of mixed roasted veggies, including eggplant, zucchini, and bell peppers
- Four ounces of crumbled goat cheese
- Two tablespoons of freshly chopped basil
To taste, add salt and pepper.
- Olive oil to pour on

Guidelines:
1. Set oven temperature to 400°F, or 200°C.
2. Using a slightly floured surface, roll out the puff pastry sheet to fit a baking sheet or tart pan. Put the pastry on the baking sheet or inside the pan.
3. To keep the pastry from puffing up too much while baking, prick it all over with a fork.
4. Evenly distribute the roasted vegetables on top of the pastry.
5. Over the vegetables, scatter the chopped basil and crumbled goat cheese.
6. To taste, add salt and pepper for seasoning.
7. Over the top, drizzle a little olive oil.
8. Bake for 25 to 30 minutes, or until the pastry is crispy and golden brown, in a preheated oven.
9. Take it out of the oven and let it a few minutes to cool down before slicing.
10. The goat cheese and roasted veggie tart can be served warm or room temperature.
11. Have fun!

Recipe #2: Goat cheese tart with caramelized onions, mushrooms, and

Information about Nutrition:
320 calories each serving
12g of protein

- 28g of carbohydrates
- 18g of fat
- One and a half hours for cooking
- Quantity Per Serving: 6 pieces

Components:
One sheet of thawed puff pastry
- Two large onions, cut thinly
- Eight ounces of chopped mushrooms
- Two teaspoons of butter
- Two tsp olive oil
- Four ounces of crumbled goat cheese
- Two tablespoons of freshly chopped thyme
To taste, add salt and pepper.

Guidelines:
1. Set oven temperature to 400°F, or 200°C.
2. Using a slightly floured surface, roll out the puff pastry sheet to fit a baking sheet or tart pan. Put the pastry on the baking sheet or inside the pan.
3. Melt the butter and olive oil in a big skillet over medium heat. Add the sliced onions and cook for 20 to 25 minutes, stirring now and then, until they are caramelized and golden brown.
4. When the mushrooms are cooked, add them to the skillet and simmer for a further five minutes.
5. Evenly cover the pastry with the caramelized onion and mushroom mixture.
6. Over the vegetables, scatter the chopped thyme and crumbled goat cheese.
7. To taste, add salt and pepper for seasoning.
8. Bake for 25 to 30 minutes, or until the pastry is crispy and golden brown, in a preheated oven.
9. Take it out of the oven and let it a few minutes to cool down before slicing.

10. Serve the goat cheese, caramelized onion, and mushroom tart warm or room temperature.
11. Have fun!

Recipe 3:

Goat Cheese Tart with Tomato, Spinach, and

Information about Nutrition:
- 280 calories each serving
- 11g of protein
- 25g of carbohydrates
- 15g of fat
– Prep Time: 60 minutes
- Quantity Per Serving: 6 pieces

Components:
One sheet of thawed puff pastry
- One cup of chopped cherry tomatoes
- Two cups of raw spinach
- Four ounces of crumbled goat cheese
- Two tablespoons of freshly chopped basil
To taste, add salt and pepper.
- Olive oil to pour on

Guidelines:
1. Set oven temperature to 400°F, or 200°C.
2. Using a slightly floured surface, roll out the puff pastry sheet to fit a baking sheet or tart pan. Put the pastry on the baking sheet or inside the pan.
3. Evenly distribute the cherry tomato halves on the pastry.
4. Across the tomatoes, distribute the young spinach leaves.
5. Over the vegetables, scatter the chopped basil and crumbled goat cheese.
6. To taste, add salt and pepper for seasoning.
7. Over the top, drizzle a little olive oil.

8. Bake for 25 to 30 minutes, or until the pastry is crispy and golden brown, in a preheated oven.

9. Take it out of the oven and let it a few minutes to cool down before slicing.

10. The goat cheese, tomato, and spinach tart can be served warm or room temperature.

11. Have fun!

Recipe 4:

Tart with Goat Cheese and Roasted Red Pepper

Information about Nutrition:
- 290 calories each serving
- 10g of protein
- 27g of carbohydrates
- 16g of fat
- One and a half hours for cooking
- Quantity Per Serving: 6 pieces

Components:
One sheet of thawed puff pastry
- Two sliced roasted red peppers
- Four ounces of crumbled goat cheese
- Two tablespoons of freshly chopped parsley
To taste, add salt and pepper.
- Olive oil to pour on

Guidelines:
1. Set oven temperature to 400°F, or 200°C.

2. Using a slightly floured surface, roll out the puff pastry sheet to fit a baking sheet or tart pan. Put the pastry on the baking sheet or inside the pan.

3. Evenly distribute the slices of roasted red pepper over the pastry.

4. Over the peppers, scatter the goat cheese crumbles and chopped parsley.

5. To taste, add salt and pepper for seasoning.

6. Over the top, drizzle a little olive oil.

7. Bake for 25 to 30 minutes, or until the pastry is crispy and golden brown, in a preheated oven.

8. Take it out of the oven and let it a few minutes to cool down before slicing.

9. Serve the tart with goat cheese and roasted red pepper warm or room temperature.

10. Have fun!

CONCLUSION

"The Complete Low Cholesterol Cookbook For Beginners UK" is an invaluable tool for people who want to make conscious dietary choices and strengthen their heart health. Because cardiovascular diseases are so common in the UK, lowering cholesterol is crucial to leading a healthy lifestyle.

This cookbook provides a wide range of mouthwatering, wholesome recipes that are especially crafted to be low in cholesterol. It makes sure that even inexperienced cooks can effortlessly navigate and prepare these dishes by offering a wide range of options to suit various tastes and dietary preferences.

People can eat delicious meals and take control of their cholesterol by using the recipes in this cookbook. A variety of components, such as whole grains, lean meats, fresh produce, and healthy fats, are used in the recipes to support a diet low in heart disease.

Furthermore, this cookbook offers more than just recipes. It provides insightful knowledge and advice on reducing cholesterol, switching out ingredients, and implementing healthier cooking methods. It provides novices with the information and resources they need to take charge of their heart health and make educated food decisions.

"The Complete Low Cholesterol Cookbook For Beginners UK" invites people to go on a culinary adventure that pleases the palate and supports heart health. With its emphasis on healthful ingredients and approachable style, this cookbook is a useful resource for anyone looking to enhance their general health with tasty and nourishing meals.

This cookbook is a great place to start if you want to control your cholesterol, avoid heart disease, or just live a healthier lifestyle. It puts novices on the path to a healthier future by providing them with the tools they need to make tasty low-cholesterol meals.

31 Days Meal Plan

Day	Breakfast	Lunch	Dinner
1	Fluffy Oatmeal Pancakes	Mediterranean Chickpea Salad	Baked Cod with Herbed Quinoa
2	Veggie Egg White Scramble	Grilled Salmon with Dill Yogurt Sauce	Ratatouille Stuffed Bell Peppers
3	Berry Chia Seed Pudding	Lemon Herb Grilled Chicken Wrap	Whole Grain Avocado Toast
4	Whole Grain Avocado Toast	Quinoa and Roasted Vegetable Salad	Turkey Meatballs in Tomato Sauce
5	Quinoa and Roasted Vegetable Salad	Baked Cod with Herbed Quinoa	Fluffy Oatmeal Pancakes
6	Lemon Herb Grilled Chicken Wrap	Ratatouille Stuffed Bell Peppers	Veggie Egg White Scramble
7	Mediterranean Chickpea Salad	Turkey Meatballs in Tomato Sauce	Berry Chia Seed Pudding
8	Grilled Salmon with Dill Yogurt Sauce	Roasted Vegetable and Goat Cheese Tart	Whole Grain Avocado Toast
9	Baked Cod with Herbed Quinoa	Fluffy Oatmeal Pancakes	Quinoa and Roasted Vegetable Salad
10	Ratatouille Stuffed Bell Peppers	Veggie Egg White Scramble	Lemon Herb Grilled Chicken Wrap

11	Turkey Meatballs in Tomato Sauce	Berry Chia Seed Pudding	Mediterranean Chickpea Salad
12	Roasted Vegetable and Goat Cheese Tart	Whole Grain Avocado Toast	Grilled Salmon with Dill Yogurt Sauce
13	Fluffy Oatmeal Pancakes	Quinoa and Roasted Vegetable Salad	Baked Cod with Herbed Quinoa
14	Veggie Egg White Scramble	Ratatouille Stuffed Bell Peppers	Lemon Herb Grilled Chicken Wrap
15	Berry Chia Seed Pudding	Turkey Meatballs in Tomato Sauce	Whole Grain Avocado Toast
16	Whole Grain Avocado Toast	Lemon Herb Grilled Chicken Wrap	Roasted Vegetable and Goat Cheese Tart
17	Quinoa and Roasted Vegetable Salad	Grilled Salmon with Dill Yogurt Sauce	Fluffy Oatmeal Pancakes
18	Lemon Herb Grilled Chicken Wrap	Baked Cod with Herbed Quinoa	Veggie Egg White Scramble
19	Mediterranean Chickpea Salad	Ratatouille Stuffed Bell Peppers	Berry Chia Seed Pudding
20	Grilled Salmon with Dill Yogurt Sauce	Turkey Meatballs in Tomato Sauce	Whole Grain Avocado Toast
21	Baked Cod with Herbed Quinoa	Roasted Vegetable and Goat Cheese Tart	Quinoa and Roasted Vegetable Salad

22	Ratatouille Stuffed Bell Peppers	Fluffy Oatmeal Pancakes	Lemon Herb Grilled Chicken Wrap
23	Turkey Meatballs in Tomato Sauce	Veggie Egg White Scramble	Mediterranean Chickpea Salad
24	Roasted Vegetable and Goat Cheese Tart	Berry Chia Seed Pudding	Grilled Salmon with Dill Yogurt Sauce
25	Fluffy Oatmeal Pancakes	Quinoa and Roasted Vegetable Salad	Baked Cod with Herbed Quinoa
26	Veggie Egg White Scramble	Lemon Herb Grilled Chicken Wrap	Ratatouille Stuffed Bell Peppers
27	Berry Chia Seed Pudding	Whole Grain Avocado Toast	Turkey Meatballs in Tomato Sauce
28	Whole Grain Avocado Toast	Quinoa and Roasted Vegetable Salad	Roasted Vegetable and Goat Cheese Tart
29	Quinoa and Roasted Vegetable Salad	Grilled Salmon with Dill Yogurt Sauce	Fluffy Oatmeal Pancakes
30	Lemon Herb Grilled Chicken Wrap	Baked Cod with Herbed Quinoa	Veggie Egg White Scramble
31	Mediterranean Chickpea Salad	Ratatouille Stuffed Bell Peppers	Berry Chia Seed Pudding